Meal Prep

The Essential Meal Prep Guide to Make Clean Eating a Natural Habit and Make Weight Loss Faster Easier and More Successful

By Jennifer Marshall

The trademarks that are used are without any consent, and the publication of the trademark is without permission or backing by the trademark owner. All trademarks and brands within this book are for clarifying purposes only and are the owned by the owners themselves, not affiliated with this document.

Table of Contents

Introduction

Hello, I'm Jennifer Marshall. I wrote this book for you in hopes that it will provide you with the information and the confidence to create an effective and reliable meal prepping routine for yourself. Setting up a consistent habit of planning and preparing meals ahead of time is so crucial to creating a sustainable diet. Our diet is literally the fuel that keeps us going in our lives. Without the proper nutrition and reliable source of consistent, healthy fuel, we are not able to perform our best and therefore will not be able to be our best possible selves every day.

Without a plan or preparation, we tend to react to each meal or snack time unconsciously, or at the very last minute. I'm sure you can see how this often leads to poor food decisions and unbalanced diets. Failing to prepare also leads to inevitably spending more money when you are away from home without a proper meal on hand. I often find that not meal planning also tends to leave me with more food that must be thrown away because it was not eaten before it had spoiled.

Most people who have mastered their health and gained the desired results in their bodies will tell you that a huge portion of their success can be attributed to their consistent commitment to meal planning and preparing their food ahead of time, for half or all of the following week. Life gets too crazy and complex to have to decide on meals as they arrive. This is true if you are only deciding on meals for yourself, or if you are responsible for feeding an entire household or family. Being prepared is the absolute key to success. It is as simple as that. And how you choose to utilize this awesome tool can be super simple or highly complex. It is completely up to you. Once you understand the knowledge and the principles, you can use them to your own advantage.

You will probably have noticed that I purposefully did not create a recipe book here. This is because I want this to be a guide book that you can use to adapt to whatever lifestyle you have and want. You will get to customize this practice in a way that best suits and benefits you personally. You are not confined to use any specific meal plan or recipes that I have chosen. There are plenty of recipe books out there that simply skim over all of the most important tools and aspects of meal prepping. This book is focused on guiding you toward building a routine that you can adapt and rely on through any of life's situations.

I am so happy to get to go on this journey with you and I hope that I am able to serve you in the best ways possible. Remember to keep an open mind and to take everything I discuss and compare it with what seems logical and doable for you.

Let's begin!

Chapter 1: What Meal Prepping Can Do for You

With a rise in the popularity of meal prepping, there is an undeniable difference in the opportunity to get more done and to be more successful in this area than we have ever known before. The resources that we have, as well as the technology allow us to use examples from other people- even videos online- to duplicate the tools and the methods used, and to get very similar results. Having meal prepping on your side can have so many benefits it can be life changing. It can have a profound effect on every area of your life. Think about it; you eat multiple times per day, every single day. The kind of foods that you are eating will dictate how you feel physically, emotionally and spiritually.

This means that your energy needed to perform anything in your everyday life depends heavily on the quality of foods you eat. And this in turn affects the dynamics of your family and your relationships. You need to rely on your diet to keep you going. Assuring that you have your meals and snacks available for quick preparation keeps you on track, even amidst the crazy, unpredictability of life.

If you can learn to use meal prepping effectively and find the right routine for your schedule, you can end up saving a ton of time in your day, and also in your week. Time during the week can often get hectic, and you need to be ready to adapt and roll with whatever might happen to come up.

Of course, better planning also leads to lower levels of stress in life. I am always interested in having lower levels of stress. How about you? Stress can be caused by panic brought on when you don't know how to handle a situation. Or perhaps when you are overwhelmed and struggle to get meals ready to eat in time. If you get the right routine down you can be more prepared for life, and have a much more enjoyable time cooking and prepping your meals. You are more likely to be able to work at a calmer pace when it comes time to make meals. And really, this is time well spent. With meal prepping, you are building a healthy habit.

A healthy habit like this can not only help to make life work more effectively, but it also gives you more confidence, self-esteem and trust in yourself to act and follow through on achieving the things that you want in your life. The more you stick to your commitments and produce positive results, the more belief you will have in what is possible to accomplish. You will be encouraged to dream big and take consistent action.

Something that makes meal preparation especially helpful is that it provides portioned-out meals on standby for whenever you need them. Keeping track of portion sizes can be a time-consuming chore, particularly if you are tracking things as you go. But preparing your meals ahead of time, at least a significant percentage of them, can make things so much easier and your results more reliable. All of these principles can be adapted and applied to meals for your whole family or household. Even with the many different preferences that they are bound to have; meal prepping can work incredibly well in a family setting. I find that using this type of planning is really useful in my family. When I plan ahead and have ingredients prepped and ready to go, I can spend less time and stress worrying over dinner, and consequently spend more time focused on my family.

The absolute same idea goes for entertaining and event planning. The more you focus your trained attention in this area ahead of time, the more thought and effective decisions can be made and executed in advance. When I am planning any event, first I want to know the date and the place it will take place. Then I want to know what I will be offering to eat and drink, and how much of it I will need to purchase and prepare, which is part of my next task- making the guest list. The sooner you do this for a party, the more successful this area of your party will be. I believe that it is super important to have enough substantial food for your guests. Prepping food for many people can be pretty daunting. Fortunately, many components can be made a few days ahead of time, and can save you a lot of last-minute hustle and worry when it comes time for your guests to start arriving.

Shopping trips will undoubtedly go smoother when you know what you need, how it will be used and when. You can cut down on unnecessary spending on impulses and uninformed decisions. Not to mention cutting down on extra trips to the grocery store. Sometimes extra shopping trips are made out of convenience, at a different store than you might do your usual shopping at- maybe one closer to your home. This can seem like a great idea- just a quick pick-up trip for a few items; no big deal just got to the nearest store that is open. Well, here you may not get the same selection or price break as your usual grocery store, and you may end up settling and getting something totally different from what you originally needed. You may need to alter your recipes, and it can definitely put extra complications into your meal plans. Plan ahead, optimize your shopping trips and you will get more control over the situation.

I mean really, the benefits are many! Would you like some more! Okay! Planning and prepping meals can also help you to infuse much more variety and possibility into your day-to-day diet. While it's true that meal prepping can be done easier during a week that contains very few different meals, it is also true that you can use this process as a way to mix up a boring eating routine. If you prep your foods in a way that allows you to mix and match ingredients, you can create multiple options for yourself, and still leave space in the week where you can be spontaneous and incorporate different variations however you want. It really doesn't have to be repetitive or monotonous, if you don't want it to be.

It is of course, a main goal in this endeavor to automate your planning, prepping and cooking routines, while allowing you to use all of your ingredients while they are still as fresh as possible. We do not want food to spoil, unused in the refrigerator, pantry or freezer. It is a total waste, a missed opportunity and completely unnecessary if planned well enough.

If you have the opportunity to get help with this process, take advantage of it because it will be a significant help. If you can enlist your family or your roommates, then that is fantastic. You can also get together with friends or family, bring your ingredients and make it a meal prepping party. We will talk more about enlisting help further along in this book.

Chapter 2: Building Your Habits and Schedule

Now, when it comes to building this new habit, I want to say first that there is no right or wrong way to do this. Your method of meal prepping will either be helpful to you, or it won't. If it isn't, there is no harm done. You can simply change up your methods and get back on track. Also, this is a very personalized habit to build, so everyone will have their own variation of a meal prep day and it will depend greatly on the individual. That being said, there are a lot of wonderful tips and hints to meal prepping that can save you a lot of time and trouble and can make your prep routine a more pleasant and successful experience. This process will help you to set up ease and automation in your meal prepping routine.

This is one of my favorite chapters because it is where you will really start planning, committing to your plans and taking action. There is nothing quite as powerful as taking the knowledge you've received and immediately putting it into action. Here is some step-by-step how-to for you. I would recommend that you start by pulling out your planner or calendar, in order to scan your schedule and find out the most optimal time to integrate this very important, new addition into your life. Choose the day that you plan to do your meal prepping on.

Try to pick a day when you will have the time to plan the week, prep food, cook and clean. Some people like to do their grocery shopping before this process, on the dame day. Others like to meal plan one day, and do their shopping and meal prepping the following day; but you can decide which you prefer better. Choose as your meal prep day, the day just before the week starts, or before the day you will need food prepared for. This will ensure you are the most stocked up and that your food will be as fresh as possible when you are ready to eat it. If you are not sure what day to do your meal prepping on, consider the following. The most helpful times to have your meals prepared for are times when you are particularly busy, or times when you will not be able to prepare a proper meal when it comes time to eat. Are there days when you will be away from home during meal times? Do you have any nights where you will be home late and will be too tired to cook? These are excellent days to have meals prepped and ready for.

Choose the days in which you will need meals for and write or type them out. Plan to do your meal prepping the day or evening before the first day of this span of time. The number of days prepared for is up to you, but most people fall on either side of two possible options. Option number one is to prep once per week, usually on a Sunday to prepare for the standard Monday through Friday week. The other option is to prep on two days, splitting the week in half, for example, on Sunday and Thursday. I would recommend preparing no more than 5 days worth of food at a time, in order to avoid food spoiling or becoming less palatable. But if you are sure that what you are preparing is a dried, non-perishable food, for example, that will stay fresh, then feel free to prepare it a bit farther in advance. Be sure to check that particular food's shelf life, if you are unsure. We will go further into food shelf lives in later chapters.

Keep in mind while planning your meal prep day that it can take roughly 1-3 hours, from start to finish. You can also split you prepping into increments of about 15 minutes or so, to chop, portion, and store food (say, for the next day). I find that I like to do my meal prepping in bulk 1-2 times per week, depending on my weekly schedule, but this incremental method can be very helpful for more perishable foods or for situations where you just can't find more than 15 minutes at a time to do your planning and prepping. This may also be great for weary, sleepy new parents of a newborn baby. These shorter sessions require smaller chunks of time and energy.

Now that you have considered your own schedule, and picked a meal prep day that works for you- mark your calendar, set a reminder, adjust your schedule and stick to it. Commit to your meal prep routine. This must stick if it's going to make a difference. If you need to readjust your day once in a while, that is perfectly fine; but your chosen day should hold the utmost importance in your weekly schedule. Commit.

Next sort out exactly which meals you need to prepare on your chosen day. And also, who will you be preparing meals in advance for- perhaps your family, parent or significant other? You may even like to pre-portion your pet's food in advance to make life easier and assure correct portions. This can work for the whole household. So for each member you are prepping for, figure out the total number of meals, snacks, etc. Consider special diets and allergies, as well as special occasions. If you need all meals, from morning to night, then plan how many breakfasts, lunches, dinners and snacks (as well as water and other drinks, if necessary). You can edit out any meals that you do not need to prep ahead of time.

Now total out your meals and snacks, and record any other information you will need to know for your weekly prep. It may help to make yourself a little chart or menu for your reference. You can record each day of the week, meal type and what you are eating. Extra points if you give each meal an approximate time of eating, to better keep that on track as well. Next decide what needs to be cooked, thawed, opened, chopped, grated, etc. Note this when planning your prep session. And remember to make this fun! Keep in mind anything that you can include to make your food prep a more enjoyable experience is worth doing. Do you want to make it a social gathering, or go all Zen and do it on your own, concentrating on the process.

It is important to decide the type of meal prepping you are going to be doing, overall. Are you going to mix-and-match meals as you go, day by day, or do you want each meal completely prepared to take and go? Let's talk about the differences between these two strategies.

Macro prepping

This type of meal prep strategy involves preparing balanced meals completely, and storing them in single-serving containers. You can just grab them and go without thinking about choosing toppings or sides very much. There is not too much combining besides perhaps dressings or other extras that are added just before eating. This is a good strategy for a really tight schedule and requires less thought when the day comes to grab that particular meal. This strategy can be more monotonous if you choose many portions of the same meal. It can also be more exciting if you plan to have more varied kinds of meals every day.

Mix-and-Match Prepping

With this method, you will leave a lot of your entrée's ingredients, sides and toppings separate in containers. You can mix them together each day in whatever combination you like. This can give you more variety and the chance to switch things up daily. In this method it is very useful to choose 2 or more different types of food group or macro (Protein, Carbohydrate, Fat, Veggie, etc.) to make. Try to balance out how many of each you will actually need each day. You may even find it helpful to make a grid for yourself, with all of your choices in each food category.

Some great examples of foods to prepare for your mix-and-match method are:

-chopped veggies and fruits you can eat with a dipping sauce or dressing; for example, carrots and cucumber with salad dressing or apples and celery with peanut butter.

-pieces of pita or tortilla for dipping in hummus, or some flat bread baked in the oven to make toasted chips for dipping.

-a mix and match salad, such as your choice of chopped lettuce, spinach, chopped chicken, hard boiled eggs, olives, tomatoes, cucumbers, sunflower seeds, and beets. You can just keep everything separate, and create a different salad each day.

-Tostadas with your choice of various proteins, vegetables and toppings

Once you've chosen how and when you are going to meal prep, the next thing to do is to shop for your appropriate ingredients and start prepping! At the end of the week and after you've enjoyed all of your meals (if you *have* enjoyed them), you can take a look at what worked and what didn't work so well. Was there anything left uneaten at the end of the week? Are you planning to eat those few lonely meals anytime soon? If not, consider perhaps not making as many of that particular meal next time. This kind of reflecting and reevaluating will help you to improve your meal prep routine each and every week, and as a result, your general nutritional game.

I hope that you grow to love your meal prepping ritual. It can be a mighty powerful tool to help you work and feel your best every day. Remember to commit to your new healthy habit before deciding to change or abandon it completely. Give it a fair chance to show you some substantial results, whether good or bad; helpful or not helpful. When you find the right routine, it can make a huge difference for you in your life.

Chapter 3: What Do You Want to Get From Meal Prepping?

When deciding to start meal prepping, it is important to really know what you are looking to achieve. Why do you want to learn how to meal prep? Set some goals for yourself and consistently work toward them. I always stress making goals and building up your "why" because it can really give you the emotion and the drive to make positive changes more effectively. What goals you set will reflect your choices, methods and ultimately the path you choose.

So why are you choosing to do this? Are you a bit overweight and need the support of a powerful foundation to get yourself into shape? Are there health reasons that propel you toward a healthier diet? Meal prepping is certainly an excellent dietary or weight loss tool to utilize. Do you perhaps have too much chaos in your life, and need more control over your meals and eating times? This is another fantastic reason to use meal planning and prepping. Some people have incredibly hectic lives and schedules and it isn't hard to imagine this kind of day-to-day life getting chaotic and off track. This can be a super structured system, or even partly structured, and you can begin to regain the power to guide your life back to where you want it to be. If you have a particular condition or allergy that requires you to have a special diet, using this type of planning can make life easier, especially if you often find yourself on-the-go and do not have the availability of foods that stay within the guidelines of your diet.

Whatever your reasons for meal prepping, you can be sure that it will help to streamline and organize your eating patterns to allow you more time and less stress-when it applies to food, anyway. It can mean the difference between failing and succeeding at times. As the saying goes, failing to plan is planning to fail. Planning and prepping gives you the power to succeed.

How and When to Multi-task

To some people, meal prepping may seem like a huge, overwhelming task. But really, it only needs to be as complicated as you want to make it. There are tons of ways you can save time, energy and even money by doing things in a more effective way. By learning when and how to multi-task, and doing things in the best possible way while leaving out the unnecessary parts, you can make your time and effort really count.

One of the first steps you should work on streamlining is your meal planning and shopping strategies. While planning your meals and making shopping lists are you writing many of the same items down each week? Could you benefit from creating or finding a meal planning template? There are s ton of free varieties online, and you can also make a customized one for yourself.

When it comes to the actual prepping, I find that already having a clean space to work in and the right tools (that are clean and in the right spot) helps me so much. This is because it makes me feel more willing to do the necessary work. Try to keep your kitchen cleaning routine consistent. This is the epicenter of your nutritional success; or failure. Well, in all honesty, I don't actually believe in failure, if you take what you've learned and move forward, but I do believe in setting yourself up for success and solving problems before they arise. Having a clean work space is practical and setting this up for your self can boost your motivation and overall productivity.

You can save quite a bit of time by creating a binder, box or folder on your computer that contains all of your recipes, conversion charts, cook times and other reference information in one spot. Obviously, the more organized you are with this, the faster you will be able to retrieve what you need, when you need it.

I would recommend keeping the following as a reference:

Measurement conversion charts

Most used recipes

Meal plan templates

Food storage and shelf life information

Freezing guidelines

Meat cooking guides

List of staple ingredients

List of staple meals and snacks

I also like to focus on recipes that contain mostly ingredients that I already own or that I can find and purchase easily. It can be complicated to try to create several recipes, that all have different ingredients. It is especially frustrating when they require difficult-to-find ingredients. However, I have to say that Amazon and similar sites will probably have most of the more obscure ingredients that you may be looking for. And don't forget about international markets. You may find that they have a great selection and discounts on some of the foods that you will need to buy. To make meal prepping manageable over a long period of time, you've got to have access to everything that you need, without substantially raising the cost of your groceries every week. Try to look for ingredients that are really versatile, that you will be able to use in many different ways.

Another way to boost your efficiency in the kitchen is to reduce the amount of mess you make as you are working. There are some pretty helpful tools and tricks you can use to keep a cleaner workspace as you prep and cook. This will allow you to spend less time cleaning up, and more time getting to enjoy the rest of your life. This is one of the most important benefits of meal prepping. Enjoy it! A great way to cut down on messes made while cooking is to use a grease guard. This is a round, screened disk with a handle that you can place over a pot or pan while cooking. It helps to reduce a lot of sauce and oil splatters on the stove, and also lessens the risk of you or anyone else being burned by hot, popping liquids. Even water can get pretty aggressive in a super hot pot or pan. Your grease guard will keep things contained while still leaving your food relatively uncovered and able to breathe; as well as be easily monitored.

I also recommend having enough dish towels, oven mitts, pot holders, trivets and cleaning towels or rags to handle any kind of situation you might need them for. When you do not have enough dish towels, you may be constantly looking for something to wipe your wet hands on or to dry off a dish you've just washed. If you do not have enough cleaning towels you may be tempted to use your dish towel for a dirtier job, which leaves you with no clean drying towel. The same goes for pot holders and oven mitts. If you don't have the proper supply, you will undoubtedly be using your dish towel or some other improvisation to grab your hot food from the stove or oven. I'm sure you can see how this can be problematic. Be prepared with some towels for drying, some for cleaning, some oven mitts and some pot holders or trivets. Trust me- it helps a lot!

When it comes to cooking, I find that is best to order your cooking and prepping in relation to cook times. Start with the food that takes the longest to cook, for example chicken, other meats and soups. Try to gauge the time it is going to take you to prepare each component of your meal preparation. If there is a food that will be simmering or baking for an extended period of time, go ahead and get that started first. That way it has time to cook and cool by the time you are ready to pack up and store everything. Once that has started cooking you can move onto the next, most time-consuming part of your meal prep. This method of ordering cooking and preparing according to time needed will keep your routine organized and take less time to get done each week. Every week that you stick to the same reliable routine, you will get better at it and it will become more natural and in turn will come with more ease and be less time-consuming. We will go into this in more detail in the chapter in which we will put all of our meal prepping steps into action.

While on the subject of saving time and effectively multi-tasking, I will say that there is the risk of over-multi-tasking. If you are getting overly stressed or getting overwhelmed you may be trying to do too much at the same time. An octopus in the kitchen comes to mind when I think about over-multi-tasking. We each have only 2 arms, at most and one brain. You want to use them strategically or you will end up undermining what you are trying to achieve.

I am hoping to help you create a meal prep habit that you can enjoy. Try to make it as fun as you can. This routine is something you want to be able to commit to doing no matter what comes up in life. So you need to make it into something you want to do. Stressing yourself out nearly defeats the purpose of meal prepping at all. So in order to lessen the stress of the process, make sure you are only doing as much as you can comfortably do at one time. Adjust your methods and your environment until you find the right situation for you. Everyone will be different in how they meal prep. Find your happy balance and stick to it.

Chapter 4: Getting the Right Nutritional Balance

In order to get the most out of your meal prepping routine, you'll want to be sure that you are aligning your meals with your health and fitness goals. If you are working on losing weight you will need to focus on getting enough proper nutrition while eating less calories than you burn in a day; consistently throughout several weeks. Take this into consideration as you plan your meals. If you are building muscle while losing fat, you will need to adjust your ratio of proteins, carbohydrates and fats respectively. I would generally say to aim for 50 % produce, 25% protein and fat and 25% carbohydrates in each meal (when those food groups are present in a meal). Whatever your current health or weight objectives are, try to include the highest quality ingredients possible that will serve your body with the greatest health benefits (while still being delicious!) That is the universal goal. Everyone wants to be healthy, right? So pay attention to what is in your food. Read the labels and judge each food, to determine if it is worth eating. If you really want to achieve your goals, this is a must.

Avoid destructive ingredients like refined sugars and processed garbage. Try to get organic when you can and include plenty of whole, fresh foods. Be sure to include healthy fats like olive oil, coconut oil, nuts, seeds and avocados. Getting enough fat in your diet helps with proper brain function, lubricates the whole body, and moisturizes your skin, hair and nails. Healthy fats also ensure that you are more satisfied with each meal, without needing to eat more and more of them. Whole food fats feel rich and luxurious when you eat them. Any healthy source of these foods will make your diet more flavorful and more substantial. Healthy foods will not feel like such a chore to eat, and you will not be craving unhealthy fats nearly as much. Overwhelming cravings for fatty, rich foods can be troublesome little monsters in your mind and body. Be sure to have a reliable stock of good, nourishing fats to combat the cravings. As long as you are including a good, balanced variety of each necessary food category, you can be assured that you are getting a healthy, balanced diet that will support you in your life; whatever that life may be.

Chapter 5: The Foods You Can Benefit From Prepping

One of the most complex aspects of meal prepping will actually be *what* you are preparing to carry you through the week. You can get a routine down, and arm yourself with the right tools and storage containers, but the important part of this process is ultimately about the food that you eat. And your time is best spent eating foods that will make you feel your best. I recommend trying to keep as close to a whole foods diet as possible- closest to natural foods. These are the most harmonious for your body. When meal prepping, you want to be sure that you are using foods that will maintain their freshness throughout the week. Some foods and produce are more vulnerable while others are heartier and lower maintenance.

In this chapter we will discuss the best foods to include in your weekly meal prep and how to assure that they will stay in their best possible condition, until you are ready to eat them. If you want the least fussy meal prep, you can choose hearty vegetables such as carrots, celery, broccoli and cauliflower to chop up and disperse into single portions. If you are using baby carrots, it is usually better to keep them in a zipper bag to help them retain their moisture.

Sometimes you can also keep them moist by storing them in a sealed storage container with other moist produce.

The first thing you may want to do for your meal prep is to wash your fruits, vegetables and herbs that you will need to use. This will make sure that they are clean and easily accessible for whatever meal requires them, whether for cooking later or enjoying them raw. Keep in mind, however, that some fruits and vegetables may be best left unwashed until they are being eaten. This is because rinsing them can tend to make them ripen faster, and they may end up going bad too quickly. Berries are the best example for this. I would only recommend pre-washing berries for the very next day- no further ahead. Tomatoes also tend to be better this way, as they ripen very quickly. I also leave off rinsing asparagus, for a longer freshness. Lettuce can be washed ahead as long as you allow it to fully dry (either by air drying or by using a salad spinner), and making sure to line its storage container with paper towels, or absorbent napkins before placing them into the refrigerator.

Most food once prepped, does best in the fridge in an airtight container. Refrigerator air tends to degrade open foods and cause them to lose their quality and flavor. I try to choose a leafy green that will stay fresh and crisp. I usually use romaine that I've washed and separated from the core completely. I also like to use kale because it can be especially robust when stored properly. And as an added bonus, you can marinate it to add a surprising amount of flavor. Another vegetable you can prepare ahead is onion. I like to either slice it into rings, or dice it into small pieces, depending on what I am using it for. This can be a life saver when you are ready to make dinner and the last thing you want to do is to chop onions. You can store it away in a sealed food container. The same goes for garlic and ginger, as long as you keep an eye on them and assure that you use them before they spoil or grow any mold. I usually prefer to leave cucumbers unwashed until I am ready to use them, but if you want sliced or speared cucumbers for the next day, you should be fine to prep them ahead. I find that they don't usually last much longer than that.

Produce like fresh soy beans, or other bite sized pieces can be portioned out into single servings and usually last a few days. As far as fruit goes, you can wash and cut all kinds ahead of time. You can portion out grapes and keep them in the fridge or in the freezer; which is a really great snack, especially during warmer weather. Fresh pineapple is also a great fruit to cut ahead, since it can be a bit time-consuming and tricky.

When you want to cook your vegetables, you have the option to blanch, steam, roast, sauté them, or use any other method you prefer. Any veggies you like to eat cooked can be prepared ahead; you may just want to reheat them later. If you are using the microwave, you may want to consider storing them in a class container as opposed to a plastic one, which does not do so well in high heat.

Roasting vegetables is an excellent cooking method to use in your routine. It helps to bring out their natural sweetness and is arguably the tastiest way to cook most vegetables. If you like to add a lot of flavorful seasoning to your meals, as I do, you can pre-measure some of your favorite seasoning combinations in order to save time and to assure that you are not over-seasoning, especially if they contain unhealthy ingredients such as salt. You can also portion out servings of oils, sauces, butter and other rich ingredients. I tend to overestimate my servings of these foods, if I do not have any real structure around my serving sizes. If this practice is not your thing, no worries, just disregard it and move on. For snacks, you may just want to portion them off into bags or containers.

Another example of an excellent food to prep ahead is oatmeal. You can cook your oatmeal traditionally, in the microwave or by letting it soak overnight to soften and expand by the morning, as with overnight oats. I will say that the overnight method works much better with rolled oats, as opposed to steel cut oats. Steel cut oats tend to stay pretty firm without the help of a hot stove to open up the oats. The type of oats you choose will depend on how you want to prepare them, their nutritional value and your personal taste. The great thing about oatmeal is that you can add very little else, or a handful of everything you have (usually remaining on the sweet side), and it is delicious. I like to add some dairy free butter, milk (I prefer soy), raisins and a little honey or brown sugar. If I have extra toppings available, I will add those as well. Sometimes I like to add chopped almonds, berries, cinnamon and a bit of fresh banana. Oatmeal is comforting, and is usually pretty gentle on the body, as it is easy to digest. This is a great on-the-go food if you store it in a mason jar and bring a spoon along with you.

Another sweet and delicious breakfast that you can prep in a batch is pancakes. Waffles are great as well. They can be a great addition to a busy schedule. You can just grab them and go. A great tip is to pop them in a toaster oven, if you have one. This heats them up and toasts them a little bit. You can find tons of recipes that make pancakes, waffles and crêpes much healthier and a lot simpler in the ingredients.

If you like muffins you can make a big batch at the beginning of the week and they tend to keep really well. Again, you can change the recipe and the flavor profiles in any way that suits you.

Cooked grains and lentils give you a great supply of healthy vehicles and fillers to complete your meals with. The best options, as far as health, will be brown rice, wild rice, quinoa and other whole, unrefined grains. There are a ton of them to choose from. I like to give mine a little bit of unflavored coconut oil or dairy free butter and seasoning. Then you can add your favorite vegetables and proteins.

And you will have yourself a delicious and complete meal. Lentils are a great way to add fiber and protein to your diet, and a little goes a long way (especially if you are working on slowly getting more fiber into your diet). Lentils are really flavorful and work well in a myriad of ways, including as a side, in casseroles and in soups.

Close relatives to lentils, of course, are beans. You may want to consider having some prepared for your week because they are an excellent source of healthy, clean protein. You can also use them to make a really tasty chili; complete with a batch of cornbread and you can enjoy it heated up for any meal of the day. Chilis are great, too, because you can set them up in a crock pot and let it cook slowly all day without having to worry too much about it.

If you're someone who likes to eat sushi, you can make your own rolls at home and it's pretty simple to accomplish. All it requires is some nori (seaweed) sheets, soft cooked rice and your favorite filling combinations. I like to keep it simple by using vegetables like cucumbers, cooked carrots and possibly some avocado, if you are going to eat it fairly quickly. You can also use cold meats like crab, imitation crab or even cooked chicken. Simply lay out your nori sheet, moisten the side you are adding to, add your rice and veggies in a row against the flat edge, and roll it up (making sure to seal the edges at the end of the roll with a bit of water. Once that is completed, you can slice them up with a wet knife blade and store them for later. This makes a healthy, fresh meal or snack for any time of day.

During your meal prep you will want to make sure that you have all of your proteins cooked and ready to incorporate into meals. This applies to any meats or meat alternatives that you prefer. If you are going to be using meat alternatives, such as tofu or veggie burgers, you can prepare them however you like. For pieces of tofu, you can marinate or season them, and either bake them, sauté and brown them or slice them up and leave them raw. For veggie burgers, I like to cook them in a pan with a little bit of oil until they are cooked through and browned on both sides. Hard boiled eggs are a fantastic protein to include in your meal prep. I make hard boiled eggs nearly every meal prep session because they are so versatile and easy to use. You can use them in salads, sandwiches, burritos or just leave them shelled and whole for a quick on-the-go snack. If you are concerned about cholesterol you can ditch the yolks and stick to the egg whites. If you like omelets, you can make them the night before so they will be ready to eat for breakfast or even lunch. Be sure to include your favorite veggies to make them extra healthy.

If you are preparing meats, there is a number of ways in which you can prepare them. They can be grilled, roasted, sautéed, baked, smoked, boiled or fried. And they can be filleted, shredded, cubed, sliced or any other way you prefer to cut your meat. Chicken breast is a popular meat to include because it tends to be healthy and really versatile. You can cook it however you like and it can be used in so many ways. If you are making chicken for the whole week, you even have the option of seasoning or marinating each portion with a different flavor so that you have more variety throughout your week. Any meat that you choose can also be marinated in the refrigerator overnight before cooking. This will not only give it extra flavor, but also help to tenderize it so it will be juicy and delicious once you cook it.

If you plan to use your marinades or sauces for later, you can easily make a large batch and store it in the refrigerator. That way you can simply add it to whatever you are cooking without having to mix up a new batch. And for any toppings, like seeds, nuts, chia and flax, you can portion them off and add them to any meal once you are ready to do so.

Prepping ahead also applies to waters and other drinks. It will make your life noticeably easier to portion them out so they are easy to grab and take with you anywhere. There are really so many other ideas that I can give you on what to meal prep, but in the interest of not overwhelming you too much information, I will stick with what we have here. By the way, if you are overwhelmed at the possibility of using all of the examples I have given you here, refer to your meal plan and pick a few foods from each group in a way that suits your dietary needs. Remember to keep it simple, especially if you are just starting out in this process. The point of meal prepping is to make life easier, as I've said before. So make it work for you and your own individual diet. Overtime, you can make it more complex, if you wish.

Chapter 6: Stocking the Kitchen with the Right Supplies

If you are going to be successful at meal prepping, there are some key supplies that you will, need to keep all of the components of the process running smoothly. I have included the tools and containers that I believe are necessary to have, as well as some of the optional items that can help to make things even easier for you.

Before you decide what to buy, take a look in your kitchen to see what you already have available for use. Do a quick assessment and toss out anything that is broken, melted, rusty or possibly stained. Once you have it paired down to items that are still in good condition, you can make a list of what needs to be purchased or replaced. While stocking up on the proper equipment, aim to do so slowly. Don't break the bank trying to overhaul your entire kitchen all at once. Focus on what is most important for you to have, and purchase those items first. Take the time to choose and invest in the right tools and containers. Focus on quality supplies that will work well and will stay in good condition for a long time. Also, be sure to shop around and online. You may be able to find the same brand or quality you are looking for at a much lower price. Once you have everything you need to meal prep, make sure to take great care of your tools and supplies;

pay attention to their proper maintenance and treat them with care. The aim is to avoid having to replace reusable items again in the near future.

Now let's talk about what you will need to have on hand. You want to make sure that you not only have enough food containers, but also that you have the right tools and dishes to use in the actual preparing and cooking. One of the two most important items to have for meal prepping are a good cutting board and a sharp knife that you love to use. You may want to have a few of each to make life easier, but I would say if nothing else, make sure you at least have one of each that you can just re-wash each time you need to use them. You will also need to have proper pots and pans as well as a baking sheet for cooking. Decide what sizes work best for you, and how many of each you want to start with. I recommend aiming to eventually have a medium sauté pan and a large one, a medium sauce pan and a large pot, and a large rectangular or round, flat baking sheet. For pots and pans it is very helpful to have matching lids, but if need be you can possibly improvise with a baking sheet as long as it will rest safely on top and hold most of the heat inside.

For prepping I find it is also important to include tools such as a vegetable peeler, can opener and a colander for rinsing and straining. You will also want to include your preference of spatulas, large spoons, whisks and similar cooking utensils. Some optional items include muffin tins and a garlic press, for easier minced garlic.

As far as dishes go, you can really mix and prepare in anything you like. However, I prefer to have a collection of glass mixing bowls in various sizes that can be stored nested in one another. They are durable and work very well for the task. My favorite brand for these is Pyrex, since they are made with great quality. It is a bonus if your mixing bowls also come with matching lids that can be used to store them in the refrigerator with. There are also plastic and metal mixing bowls like this available, but I find the glass just tends to work better for me. Also available are bake and store containers that are made of glass. These are like deep various-sized casserole or baking dishes that come with lids. After they have cooked and cooled, you simply add the lids and store them in the fridge. Once you have all of your cooking and prepping necessities, you will need to consider the best food storage options for you and your household. Be sure to include containers in various sizes that will be appropriate for each type of meal and ingredient.

Ultimately, you will have to decide which sized containers you need and how many to have in stock, but here are some basic guidelines for what containers work best for which foods. For storing salads, aim to have containers that are roughly 2 liters, or 64 ounces. For lunches, dinners and other main meals, 24 ounce to 34 ounce (or 1 liter) containers will work well. 4 ounce to 12 ounce containers work great for fruits and snacks, and 1 ounce containers are best for nuts, seeds, dried fruit and dressings. The shape of your containers is really your choice; just make sure that they can stack easily in the refrigerator. You may also want to consider using bento boxes or sectional containers. They might end up being a great meal prep addition for your lifestyle.

Aim for containers with air tight lids, especially for wet ingredients and dressings. It is also important to assure that your containers are made from the safest plastics possible. Aim to use containers that are safe for the refrigerator, freezer, dish washer and are BPA-free. Make it a habit not to heat any of its contents in the microwave; this can heat the plastic and possibly release harmful chemicals into your food. If you can, transfer the food into a microwave-safe dish to heat. If this isn't possible and you still need to heat your meal, keep the timing as short as possible (less than one minute). As far as safety from possible chemicals goes, glass and stainless steel containers are a healthier option, but not mandatory. I still find that plastics are more convenient, especially on-the-go. As long as you treat them with care, there is very little health risk in using them. I find it more important to limit the amount of chemicals in the actual foods I am eating; added by food manufacturers. If you want to use glass food containers, look for those with a plastic lid that has secure snaps on each side. And use an insulated lunch bag, to insure that they are well padded and protected. There are also glass containers available with silicone shells that make them less prone to being broken. I have this type of glass and silicone combination for my drinking bottles.

Most avid meal preppers will recommend using mason jars for weekly meals and I would have to agree. They are excellent for storing green salads, bean salads, fruit salads, sauces, marinades and oatmeal. To save a little extra money, feel free to repurpose food jars as well, such as ones used for pasta sauce, jellies or other sauce jars. Keep in mind, that if you want to use any jar for a single portion of food, it should be easy to eat out of with a spoon or fork.

As a side note, I will also say that zipper sandwich bags are super helpful. You can get them in sandwich and snack sizes, for single portions. You can use quart or larger sizes for bigger portions or for the freezer.

Here I will discuss some of the extras you might want to have available in the kitchen. The first extra I would almost categorize as a necessity is a stock of paper towels. These are really helpful for lining containers for clean, chopped vegetable and leafy greens. They can also be used for dabbing moisture from foods like rinsed greens and water-packed tofu. Another extra that I think is pretty important is a set of food labels. Label Once are my absolute favorite brand, because you literally only have to label each container once. Instead of disintegrating when they are wet, Label Once labels have a more glossy finish so they are very durable. They come with a fine permanent marker and a permanent pen eraser. You can also use any permanent ink to write your labels but I like the fine tip so you are able to write more clearly and fit more on the label. If you need to remove a label or if the edges start to curl up a little, these are super easy to peel off clean and replace as needed. I like to keep my pen and eraser in a cup in the kitchen where I can access them easily as I switch out container contents. Another optional tool is a salad spinner. This can be really helpful if you have a lot of leafy greens to rinse and you want to be able to quickly store them or use them in a meal. Lettuce and other leafy greens tend to stay freshest when they are stored without any extra moisture.

If you don't have a crock pot (or slow cooker) already, it may be something that you'll want to invest in, in the future. It can make certain recipes such as soups, chilis, pasta dishes, meat dishes and casserole fillings much easier to cook. In most cases, you can simply fill it up with the ingredients that your recipe calls for, set the timer and leave it to cook itself until it is ready to be eaten or stored for later. Also, you might want to consider investing in a combination rice and veggie steamer (Instant Pot is one of the most popular versions). This machine allows you to cut down on your cooking time, by combining tasks. You can steam your grains in the main compartment, and there is a top shelf basket where you can steam your vegetables and many other foods. Again, these appliances are completely optional so you can decide if they are something you want to have in your meal prepping arsenal. And lastly, a food scale might be a good investment if you are on a stricter or more exact diet and you need to know your calories, macros and precise serving sizes.

Now that you know what tools, containers and supplies you will need, and what items I recommend, you can make more informed decisions while stocking up your kitchen. This will help you to make it the best possible environment for your meal prepping routine. Take inventory of what you already have, and slowly fill in anything else that you feel will compliment your routine.

Chapter 7: Cooking and Prepping It All

Now you should know what you plan to prepare. You have your meal prep day planned, you've shopped for all of the food you'll need and you have your tools and containers ready. Next it is time to begin your meal prep. This is really where the rubber meets the road, so to speak. It works best to have a meal prep plan of action with you; either written or typed out, so you know exactly what needs to be made, and how much you need to prepare for the coming week. If you are using any specific recipes, be sure to have them close at hand. I find it works well to have each recipe printed and in a clear sheet protector, so it doesn't get any water or other ingredients on it. It can also be helpful to scan cookbook pages. Print them out and place them is a sheet protector. But if you prefer to work straight from a cookbook, or to use your own recipe method, feel free to do so.

Next you will want to pull out anything that needs to be defrosted from the freezer. You can place it in the clean sink to defrost as you are preparing everything that needs to be cooked. Another way to defrost food is to leave it in the fridge overnight, depending on what you are defrosting. Some foods can be cooked straight from the freezer, as well. Keep in mind that you will want to make enough food to fill at least 75% of your weekly meals, ideally, but you can really make the proper amount for your needs and comfort level. If you need any extra recipes or inspiration, Pinterest is an excellent resource, and I would also recommend allrecipes.com as well. This site is especially helpful if you have any extra ingredients that you aren't sure what to do with. You can type in specific ingredients to find recipes that call for them. Usually you would want to refer to these sites during your weekly meal planning session, but sometimes you may need to adjust your meals a little bit as you are prepping, especially while you are becoming accustomed to your routine. These are just some quick, helpful resources to have available in case any unexpected changes need to be made.

While you are thawing any foods that are frozen, you can preheat the oven if you are using it. Also, line your baking pans with aluminum foil or cooking oil spray before seasoning and cooking your food. This will insure easier clean up and prevent food from sticking and becoming broken into pieces. If you are cooking on the stove, try to use nonstick pots and pans so you won't have to add a lot of extra oil to your recipe. It is useful to cook up all of your proteins at once, such as making a batch of burgers (beef, turkey, veggie or otherwise) on the stove or grill while chicken breasts, or any other protein is cooking in the oven. You can also bake sweet potatoes or squash in the oven while chicken breasts are baking, if that will not affect the cooking consistency of your chicken. Most ovens are quite different, so you may want to try this out in yours to see if you can still get the right cook from the same amount of time with multiple foods baking at the same temperature. Using these methods will help you to get some of the bigger tasks out of the way first, so your meal prep will get easier and take less time as you move forward. Keep in mind that any specific foods mentioned here are merely examples and can be adapted for your own meal prep and dietary requirements.

Once you have begun cooking your food, you can organize your Tupperware or any storage containers you will be using on a counter or table top by day, so that as things finish cooking and cooling, you can begin portioning them out.

If you are going to make rice, oatmeal, cooked veggies, legumes or any foods with similar cook times or methods, you can start cooking them now. If you haven't done so already, you can also peel your potatoes and get them cooking, or skip the peeling and puncture them all over and bake or microwave them.

After your cooked food has cooled, it may still need to be prepped further. If needed, you can pull meat from the bone, chop, slice, shred, etc. If anything needs to be seasoned or have toppings added, now is a good time to do so. Once everything that requires cooking has been cooled, prepped and put into containers, you can close the lids, stack them and store them in the refrigerator.

Now that you are finished with the actual cooking, I would recommend filling the sink or a dish tub with hot soapy water and soaking any dirty dishes so they will be much easier to wash once you are done with the rest of your meal prepping. The rest of this process should be relatively easy; not to mention that the kitchen should start to cool down a little, as well. Now you should only have to do tasks such as washing fruits and vegetables, cutting things into pieces and assembling meals and snacks.

If you are preparing salads, you can assemble the ingredients in a container or a mason jar. You can either add your salad dressing to the bottom of your container, or keep it in a small container or jar on the side. In a Mason jar salad, it is best to place the wettest and heaviest ingredients on the bottom and proceed to add lighter ingredients as you go further up to the top. You can also use a similar method for bean salads as well as for oatmeal.

A helpful tip that I always like to use in my meal prep routine is to chop most of my vegetables so they are ready to use for any snack or cooked dish. This gives you a nice batch of crudités that is really versatile. It works well for chopped broccoli, cauliflower, carrots, celery and any other hearty, raw vegetable. Broccoli and cauliflower can be cut into bite-sized florets and most other veggies like celery and carrots can be cut into short spears. During this process, also be sure to wash and prepare your leafy greens. Lettuce can be pulled from the stalk leaf by leaf and placed in an airtight container. Kale can be stemmed, rolled up and thinly sliced so it makes pasta-like strips. Be sure to line your containers for all vegetables with paper towels or absorbent napkins to cut down on moisture, therefore helping them to stay fresh for longer. Nobody likes soggy, limp vegetables.

Something else that you can prepare is smoothie bags, if you enjoy having smoothies. Just take a plastic sealable bag and fill it with all of your ingredients. Squeeze all of the air out, and place each bag in the freezer. When you are ready to blend it up, simply pull out the bag, let it thaw for a few minutes on the counter, and add it to the blender. Add to this mixture a cup of your favorite milk or water, and any other of your favorite toppings such as nut butter, protein powder, chia seeds or ground flax.

Apple slices are another excellent snack to pack, for when you are busy and you want something fresh and sweet. They tend to turn brown over time so a great trick to keep them fresh is to squeeze some lemon juice over them. This also gives them a little tartness. I like to add a bit of cinnamon, as well, and sometimes eat them with a side of nut butter in a container for dipping.

Lastly, you'll want to complete your meal prepping session by insuring you have enough water ready for every day of the week. Hydration is incredibly important! You can prepare several reusable bottles and if you like, fill a pitcher with water and keep it in the fridge. You can sprinkle in any additions to flavor your water however you would like. Some great examples are lemon, mint, rosemary, strawberry and cayenne pepper.

Once everything is finished, you can begin to clean up. It may not be the most fun part of your meal prep process, but is much better to take care of it as soon as you are done working in the kitchen. So let's talk about how to make your clean up as efficient and as painless as possible.

There are a few different ways that you can handle the clean up job after you've finished your meal prep. You can choose to clean up most of the mess as you cook, or you can leave everything until the end of your prep session. Whichever method you choose, I would recommend filling the sink, or a wash tub with warm or hot soapy water, so that any dirty dishes or tools can soak until they are ready to be washed. If you prefer to leave all of the dishes and cleaning until the very end, you can simply toss all of your dishes and tools into the sink (as long as they can be submerged in water), as you dirty them. Once you are ready to wash the dishes, you can load them into the dishwasher, or wash them by hand.

Next you can tidy, spray and wipe down all counters, tables or whatever else has gotten dirty while you were cooking. If you like the process of cleaning as you go, you can still soak dishes while they wait to be washed. The difference with this process, however, is that you will be using the wait time that comes between cooking tasks to clean up your working area. This includes washing any dishes, spraying and wiping counters and putting any loose items or ingredients away. You can also use this time to wipe down any other surfaces where food has dropped or splashed, such as appliances, walls or cupboard doors. Whether you use the clean-as-you-go process or the clean-after-the-storm process, I would recommend leaving any floor sweeping or mopping until everything else is completely finished. That way you won't have to end up repeating this step several times as things have fallen to the floor. Whatever method of cleaning ends up working better for you, once you get it down, it will make your meal prepping routine go more smoothly and will even be more rewarding for you.

Chapter 8: Caution, Safety and Avoiding Mistakes

Now that you have a better idea of the meal prepping process, you can begin to put it into action and create it to become whatever you like. In this chapter we will discuss some of the extra tips that will help you to avoid many common mistakes. As you are getting used to the process of meal prepping, it is important to slowly build the habit and to build a system in your house that will allow you to learn just how much food is needed to be prepared. Be aware of making too much food ahead of time. This can cause uneaten food to go bad, or even just sacrifice the freshness and flavor because you will not be able to eat it soon enough. Once you get this part regulated and you are able to make the proper amount of food, you will not have to worry so much that any of the food you prepare will spoil. After you have been meal planning and prepping for a while, notice any foods or meals that you are eating repeatedly, every week, and you can write these down as some of your staple foods. These are foods you can repurchase consistently and count on to help get you through most weeks. This will also be a great help when you are trying to come up with possible ideas during your meal planning session. Excellent examples of these staple foods are chopped vegetable crudités like broccoli and carrots, or homemade trail mix that you never seem to get bored of. I also like to keep hard boiled eggs, oatmeal and rice on hand most of the time. And always remember, meal planning and prepping are much easier the more repeat meals you are willing to eat throughout the week.

Now as far as your routine goes, it is incredibly important that you can commit to your meal plan and prep days every single week. These habits you are building will set you up for success during the week, and it should not be taken lightly or be put off or moved around repeatedly. However, if something big comes up and by chance you aren't able to do your planning or prepping on your chosen day, then just do the best you can to stay on track. Try to get at least half, if not more of it done on your normal day; or complete the quickest, easiest prep tasks done and finish the rest on the following day. If you can, have everything you need to eat for the next day finished, so you are ready when that morning comes.

A great cooking tip that you should keep in mind is to make sure that if you are cooking meat or vegetables, they are cut into similar-sized pieces. This will allow them to cook at approximately the same time, and you will not have to babysit each individual piece as closely.

When you store your meals, avoid just mixing everything together in the same container; separate items that have different textures and levels of moisture. Mixing them all together may lead to less than appetizing textures and flavors when you go to eat your food. Also, keep foods with their own distinct flavors separate, especially foods that have very strong flavors. Let them maintain their own properties and flavors; once you are ready to eat them, then you can mix them if you wish. Another great storage tip is to look for clear plastic and glass containers, as they allow you, not only see the contents better, but also to keep an eye on each item to assure they are maintaining their best freshness and color. This is especially important if you are not using food labels to write your container's contents and prepare dates.

For times when you are on-the-go try to keep instant, easy-to-grab snacks and extras on hand for times when you won't have the chance to have a sit down meal. Things like protein bars, pretzels, trail mix and fresh fruits & veggies are great examples.

In the kitchen most appliances can be stored away in cupboards, in the pantry or on shelves when not in use. This will allow you to have more clear counter space to work on. However, if there are appliances that you use very often or daily, you may want to find a special spot on a counter or table top, next to a power outlet.

If you are in the kitchen and you find that your knife has become dull and not cutting as well, you will need to sharpen it up. If you don't have a knife sharpener handy, however, there is an easy solution. You can simply flip over a ceramic coffee cup and use the bottom rough edge to run the sides of your blade along. It will be sharpened as good as new.

During your food prep, you may find that the kitchen has been filled with various food aromas, or perhaps has even been filled with greasy, smoky smells. To cut down on unpleasant food smells, you can set a bowl of white vinegar near your cooking area before hand and it will help to absorb most of the smells. Once you are finished and the kitchen is refreshed, simply toss the vinegar down the sink and wash the bowl. If it gets too smoky in the kitchen, be sure to ventilate the room by turning on the fan and opening the windows or doors.

When working in the kitchen always choose safety over productivity and speed. You may want to rush through your meal prep to get everything done quickly, but above all you want to make sure that you are being safe and doing everything the proper way. Always remember to wear oven mitts when they are needed and use careful attention and the safest practices when you are using a knife or any kind of slicer, peeler or grater. And always make sure to keep appliances and cords out of water that may be sitting on counter tops (especially common with counters that are closest to the sink). Getting these wet may lead to electrocution or damaging the appliance.

And lastly, be sure to use the right cleaning products on your particular counters, cupboards and appliance finishes. Do not use bleach on marble or granite counter tops, or abrasive sponges on touchy surfaces or stainless steel appliances. They can get scratched or damaged, and will not look as well as before. Most surfaces will be fine with just some soapy water, a gentle sponge and a towel to buff the surface dry with. Find out which of this advice works best for you, and add it to your regular routine.

Cooking and food safety is obviously an important factor to take into account when preparing meals. But this goes beyond preventing burns, knife injuries and chicken juice contamination. There are specific guidelines when it comes to the shelf lives of food, and preventing getting sick from eating spoiled ingredients. You also want to make sure that your meals are not getting freezer burned, or sitting in unhealthy temperatures for too long. Also important is assuring that your meat is cooked thoroughly and has reached the proper heating range for consumption. In this section, we will cover the basic guidelines to help you insure your food is safe to eat and that it will taste its freshest up until the time you are ready to eat it.

The first thing that I really want to stress, and I've mentioned this before, is that you label and date your meal and snack containers. It can be really difficult to know just what is in every single storage container if you are not labeling, and it is even more difficult to know how long it is been in there if it doesn't have a date. In the refrigerator, foods will only keep so long before they begin to degrade and spoil (or grow fuzzy mold). There are many ways you can do this and it is fairly simple.

Fresh prepared foods should only be kept in the refrigerator for no more than 4 or 5 days. Some individual ingredients can last up to 1 week in the refrigerator. For grains like brown rice and oatmeal, they can last in the refrigerator for about 4 days, per batch. Large batches of sauces, marinades and dressings can be kept in the fridge for up to 1 week, and up to 3 months in the freezer. So if you make a large batch, I would recommend refrigerating half and freezing the other half. Most foods, when frozen, can keep up to a few months with no problem, as long as they are in a sealed bag or container with very little air.

For this next set of advice, you may want to have a meat thermometer available while you cook, to ensure food reaches and remains in a safe temperature before eating. And avoid leaving foods out (especially meats and dairy products) in unsafe temperatures for too long.

It is safe to leave food out for up to 12 hours, if it remains at 42°, or lower. Degrees 42°-145° are considered to be in the "danger zone". Left for too long in these conditions, food can begin to spoil and grow bacteria. Meats can withstand temperatures from 32°to 42° for up to 48 hours, properly sealed. In order to freeze meats and other foods, they must reach a maximum of 32°.

Here I have included a cooking temperature chart for meat and other foods that require specific heating temperatures.

Beef/Steak	
Rare	120°-125°
Medium-rare	130°-135°
Medium	140°-145°
Medium-well	150°-155°
Well-done	160°
Lamb	
Rare	135°
Medium-rare	140°
Medium	160°
Well-done	165°
Chicken	
Standard cook	165°

Turkey	
Standard cook	165°
Pork	
Standard cook	145°
Ham fully cooked and reheated	140°
Ground Poultry	165°
Ground Beef	160°
Eggs & Egg Dishes	160°
Casseroles	160°
Stuffing, Dressing	165°
Reheated Leftovers (with meat)	165°
Holding temperature for cooked foods	140°

Conclusion

I'd like to thank you, sincerely for taking the time to read my book. I honestly believe in the powerful results that come from the commitment to meal prep regularly. I think that in many cases, we tend to prepare and eat food on autopilot, or unconsciously in a way that undermines our wishes for how healthy we want to be in our lives. There seems to be a huge disconnect between where we want to be and the habits that we perform, or neglect day after day. Having a clear view of where you ultimately want to be is one of the first steps you can take toward closing that gap. You've got to have powerful enough reasons behind why you want it, and really build a strong foundation with the right plan, routines and individual habits.

It is my deepest hope that this book has allowed you to simplify the process, as well as to demystify any confusion you may have had about meal planning and prepping. I created this book to be very practical and straight forward, and to give you the proper tools without merely being accessories to a half-hearted recipe book. I want to provide you with the ability to take this knowledge and adapt it to your personal dietary style and needs. And with the assistance of this book, you will be able to choose recipes that will work well not only for meal prepping, but also for your personal tastes and goals. The guidelines in this book have given you a structure on which to build your personalized dietary lifestyle.

From here, you can really take it anywhere you like, whether your focus is to get healthier, lose weight, bulk up or simply to make life a little easier and less stressful. Remember to take the lessons in this book step-by-step, and if I have included anything that doesn't fit into your wants or lifestyle, than you can simply leave it out. And if you ever need to be reminded of any of the information I have covered here, you can always come back to it and refresh what you've learned. Again, thank you so much and I feel honored to have been able to share my knowledge and extensive research with you.

Deepest regards,

Jennifer Marshall

I Would Love To Hear From You!

Please feel free to send me an email with any of your questions. I am always glad to help you further your understanding of health and nutrition, and how to make it practical in your own life.

You can contact me at:
Cleverdaydream@gmail.com

References

https://www.prevention.com/food/easy-meal-prep-ideas/slide/8

http://www.mealprephaven.com/blog-1/2015/9/21/meal-prepping-101-for-beginners

http://www.thirtyhandmadedays.com/100-meal-prep-ideas/

https://mealpreponfleek.com/meal-prep-101-for-beginners/

https://www.kaylaitsines.com/blogs/lifestyle/18903859-meal-prep-101-for-beginners

https://www.beachbodyondemand.com/blog/meal-prep-101-a-beginners-guide-to-meal-prep

http://www.superfoodslife.com/meal-prep-101/

http://getinspiredeveryday.com/lifestyle/food-prep-101/

http://motivenutrition.com/meal-prep-101-tips-for-beginners/

https://www.acefitness.org/acefit/healthy-living-article/60/5466/meal-prepping-101/

https://www.kaiafit.com/meal-prepping-101

http://happyisthenewhealthy.tumblr.com/mealprep101

https://www.thespruce.com/meat-temp-chart-and-safety-tips-3056800

Leave a review!

Finally, if you enjoyed this book, then I'd like to ask you for a favor, would you be kind enough to leave a review for this book on Amazon? It helps me out a lot, and it'd be greatly appreciated!

Visit this book's page on Amazon to leave a review

https://www.amazon.com/dp/B072TV18XF

Thank you and Best of Luck to You!

More Great Titles By Jennifer Marshall!!

Below you'll find some of my other books that are popular on Amazon and Kindle as well. Simply click on the links below to check them out. I greatly appreciate it!

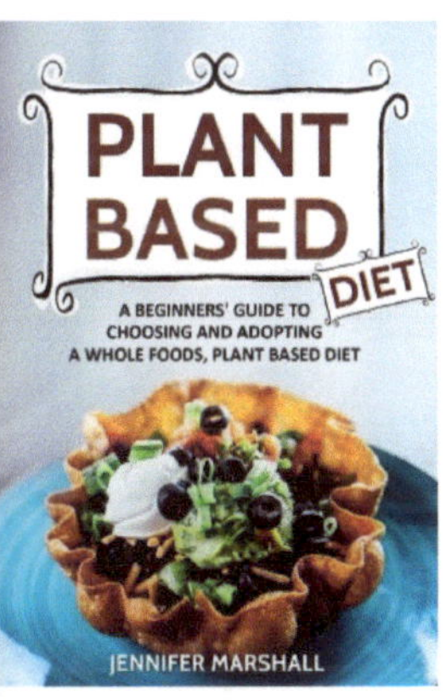

https://www.amazon.com/dp/B074SGK7K1

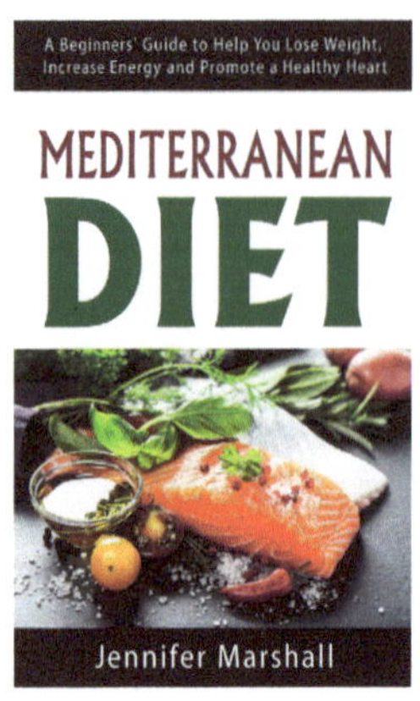

https://www.amazon.com/dp/B01M61E7H5

If the links do not work, for whatever reason, you can simply search for these titles on the Amazon website to find them.

Keep Growing. And Loving.